The Caregiver's Guide
For All Long Term Illnesses

The Caregiver's Guide For All Long Term Illnesses

Bette Thomas

iUniverse, Inc.

New York Lincoln Shanghai

The Caregiver's Guide For All Long Term Illnesses

iUniverse books may be ordered through booksellers or by contacting:

iUniverse
2021 Pine Lake Road, Suite 100
Lincoln, NE 68512
www.iuniverse.com
1-800-Authors (1-800-288-4677)

The information, ideas, and suggestions in this book are not intended as a substitute for professional medical advice. Before following any suggestions contained in this book, you should consult your personal physician. Neither the author nor the publisher shall be liable or responsible for any loss or damage allegedly arising as a consequence of your use or application of any information or suggestions in this book.

ISBN-13: 978-0-595-42617-1 (pbk)
ISBN-13: 978-0-595-86945-9 (ebk)
ISBN-10: 0-595-42617-4 (pbk)
ISBN-10: 0-595-86945-9 (ebk)

Printed in the United States of America

This book is dedicated to my wonderful husband, Chuck, who battled Parkinson's Disease for 31 years.

Watching him fight to beat Parkinson's, I realized that he needed more from me than just his pills. His strength and determination just made me more proud of his ability to continue to go on with his life.

Throughout his life, he was an example of what patients could do to improve their lives. He always had a smile and greeted others with words of encouragement.

He was truly an inspiration to all persons he came in contact with.

A SPECIAL THANKS TO:

The Lexington Area Parkinson's Disease Support Groups. Your encouragement and support are greatly appreciated.

Contents

THE CAREGIVER'S GUIDE:

For All Long Term Illnesses

Author : Bette H. Thomas

1

Introduction

This book is intended to help caregivers with the daily struggles with many diseases that patients have for a long time. Parkinson's Disease, Alzheimer's, Lou Gehrig's, and Multiple Sclerosis just happen to be a few that fit this description. Please remember that not everything suggested will help everyone. Therefore you must pick and choose the ones that you feel will help the most for your patient.

No matter which disease your patient has, it is important that you, as a caregiver, learn everything you can about that illness. This will help you understand the disease and its limitations. The uniqueness of these and other diseases is that they all begin in various ways. Your goal is to have your patient live an enjoyable life beyond the expected length of time of the disease. Your job will be easier and more enjoyable because it will enable you to do many things that you thought were impossible to help your patient.

2

Caregiver's Challenge

You and your patient are without a doubt devastated by the diagnosis your Doctor has just given you. After the disbelief begins to wear thin, you as a caregiver are thinking about what to do next. This process takes weeks and sometimes years to come to the realization that the Doctor was right.

The first thing you need to do is to have a plan of action regarding what to do about the diagnosis you have been given. The choice is one of two options you can choose. This choice must be made by the patient and caregiver together. You can refuse to believe the diagnosis and just sulk around feeling sorry for yourself, or decide to put the disease in the background and go about your business. You do not forget the disease but make some adjustments and continue with your hopes and dreams of trips to take, being with friends, and enjoying activities you like. Life goes on and it is time to set your goals and move on with your lives.

The disease is not the end of the road, but rather the beginning of a new road. The patient becomes the focus of the family of caregivers. Nurturing the patients needs, but not pitying them is of the utmost importance.

The caregiver should join a Support Group that will be able to help you understand the many variations of the patient's illness. This is an excellent way to vent frustrations you are facing and share your hopes and dreams with others.

The caregiver job is the toughest job you will ever have, but the most rewarding to know that you have enabled your patient to have a wonderful life in spite of the disease he/she is faced with. You will need help from time to time and I will offer some reasonable solutions to most of the daily problems further in this Guide Book.

3

Taking Care of Yourself

Being a caregiver, you are on demand 24 hours/7 days a week. Therefore, you need to take very good care of yourself. Be sure you eat balanced meals and get plenty of rest. There will be times when you need to get away for a few hours or even a day. This job of caregiving you have taken on is very stressful and can take a toll on you.

Don't feel as thou you are abandoning your patient. Far from that; you will be a better caregiver having been able to spend some time doing things that you enjoy. Take time to pamper yourself!

If you need help to be able to get away, contact your local home health agency, a family member, or a friend. Some senior citizens groups may be able to provide a few hours of respite care. There are adult day care centers which do a wonderful job of providing exercises, meals, crafts, and games for the patient.

4

Independence for the Patient

In this chapter, I will offer suggestions that you can use to help your patient become more independent and thereby relieve you from many tedious tasks.

4.1 Security and Safety

Move furniture to leave open space for the patient to get around safely. This should be done in all rooms. Place grab bars in the bathroom and kitchen. See your attorney to have a Living Will and Advanced Directives drawn up to your specifications. Put a copy of these in the glove compartment of your vehicle in case of an emergency. Carry a First Aid Kit in your vehicle and be sure to include rubber gloves. Remove all guns and other weapons from the patient's home. Call a family member and have them keep them. This will be very important should the patient have hallucinations. To the patient, these are very real and he/she may mistake you for a burglar or an enemy.

4.2 Clothing Needs

Buy tee shirts or blouses one size larger than he/she wears. They will be able to put these on by themselves. Get soft socks that stretch. Be sure to put socks on before pants or slacks. Buy elastic belts for men. Purchase shoes that have Velcro instead of laces. If you have good shoes with laces, you can replace the laces with corkscrew elastic shoelaces. You can purchase pull-on pants with elastic all the way around the waistband. These can be used as dress pants. Sweat pants are also useful and the same style. When buying coats or jackets, be sure they have a silky or nylon lining, especially in the sleeves. Get the patient mittens instead of gloves. They are much easier to put on their hands. A terry cloth robe is a much needed item for them. It will help them dry off after a shower and serves the purpose of allowing the patient a rest period before having to dress.

4.3 Eating Aids

When eating becomes a problem, serve as many finger foods as possible. Give the patient a spoon to eat things like peas or any other difficult vegetable. Continue to go out to eat. Let your waiter or waitress know that your patient needs to have the meat cut in small pieces. Resturants are happy to cut the meat before serving it to the patients. Drinking soup from a mug is easier for them to manage. Use only non-breakable glassware and dishes to prevent an unfortunate accident. Aladin plastic mugs with a handle and a lid are great and will avoid large spills.

4.4 Bedding

Purchase a bed bar for the patient's bed. This helps them get up from the bed and allows them to have support when standing. Get a waterproof cover for the mattress. It is like a pillow case with a zipper on the short end. Satin sheets are a must have because they help the patient move about on the bed and roll over alone.

4.5 Personal Needs

Always encourage your patient to do as much as possible on their own. It will probably take them a lot longer to do a task, but it is important that you allow them to try . Give them praise when they are finished. Continue to visit friends, go to the mall, and anywhere you want. Being around people will help keep socializing active. You need to purchase a gait belt to help you get the patient up when a fall occurs. Walkers and canes can be purchased at any medical store. If the patient needs these items they can be purchased through medicare. Check with your state medicare office for rules and guidelines. There is a door-stop alarm that can be purchased for use when the patient begins to wander out of the house at night. It has a very loud alarm and is inexpensive. It is also handy to have when traveling and staying in motels. Always carry their medication list and yours. The caregiver needs to keep these. It is also a good idea to up-date the medications list before seeing his/her Doctor. Include your patient's name, address, birthdate, phone number, and the name of the illness. When you list the medication be sure to include milligrams and times taken. At the bottom of that page, list any problems you have noticed, suggestions or concerns you may have. The caregiver should purchase an ID tag, necklace, or bracelet for the patient. It should have his/her name, address, phone number, and the illness engraved on it. Most of the items mentioned can be purchased on computers with internet access. The Doctors name and phone number can also be put on the ID tag.

4.6 Medical Equipment

As I stated in section 4.5 regarding some of the items needed for the patient, I have some of them pictured in this section. Keep in mind that you may not need all of the suggestions of medical equipment. Since this Guide Book is covering several long term illnesses, you must pick and choose the proper ones for your patient.

Suggestions regarding Medical Equipment are shown on the next few pages. Keep in mind that these are examples only as there are many styles and kinds of each. There will be times that the therapy for you to relieve your stress would be to write poetry, paint a picture, or keep a journal. These are wonderful ways to transfer your thoughts and feelings from you to paper. Of course there are several medians that can serve as a release for you. I will share with you a few poems I wrote when the going got me completely stressed out.

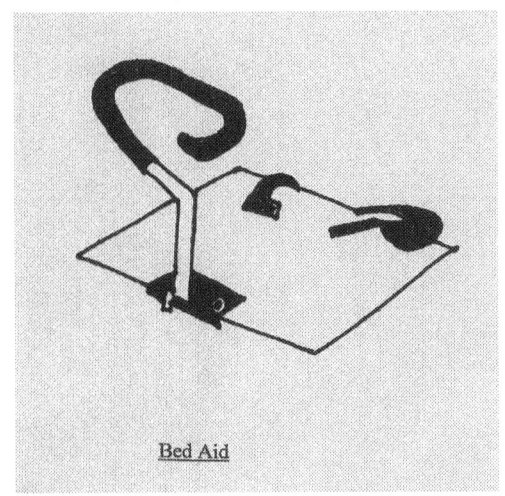

Bed Aid

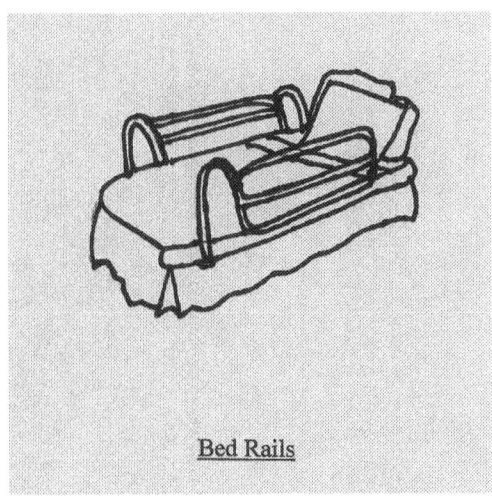

Bed Rails

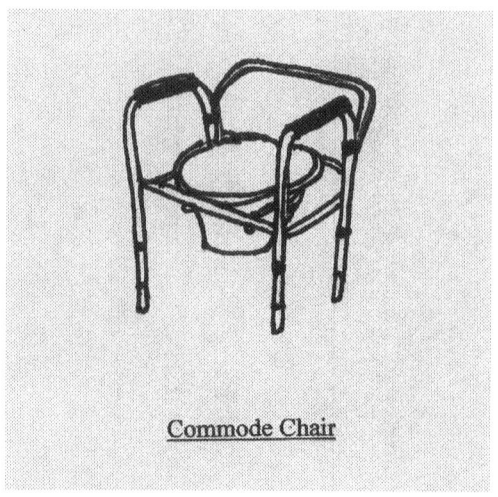

Commode Chair

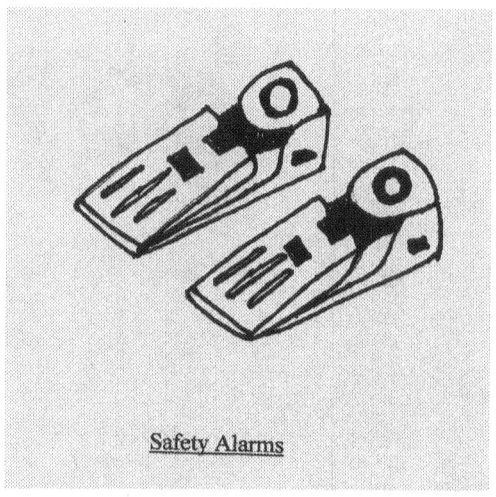

Safety Alarms

ID Tag

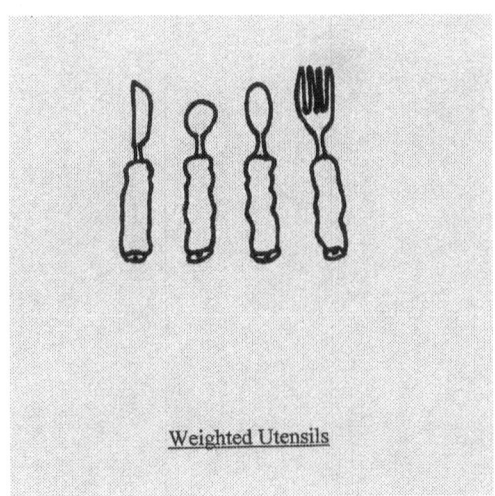

Weighted Utensils

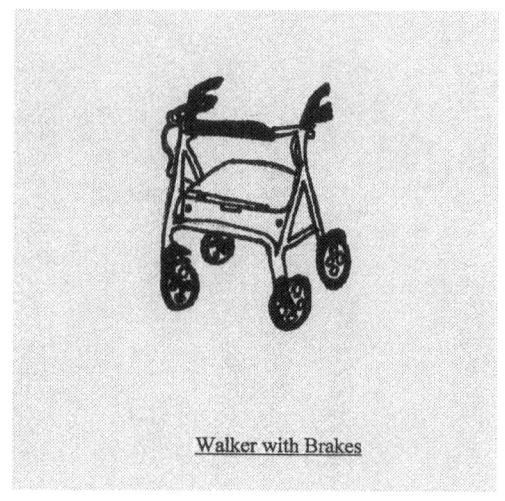

Walker with Brakes

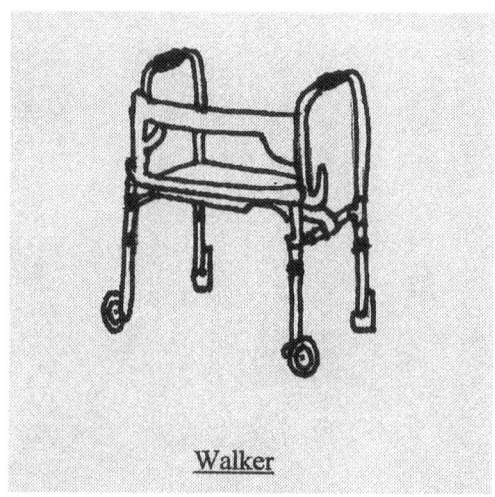

Walker

A Precious Rose

A rose is a symbol of the beauty in our lives.
Colorful, velvety, and some in stripes
It unfurls from its tiny, tight bloom,
Slowly and majestically stretching tall towards the moon.

As I gaze with awe at its glorious tints,
I suddenly get a whiff of its perfumey scents.
From its Earthly beginning to its velvety petals,
Every inch symbolic as are its ribbons and metals.

A caregiver gives it nourishment and care,
Protecting and shielding it from winter's wear.
And then as spring approaches,
The thorns of life begins its encroachment.

Each tiny thorn representing lifes hurdles.
We struggle to climb one only to find another.
But comes with each hurdle the strength and courage,
To master them all and not get discouraged.

When we complete life's journey to reach the top,
We find life's reward in the beauty that won't stop.
Enjoy each petal as nature knows,
By touching, smelling, and enjoying the beauty of this
          Precious Rose!
Written by Bette Thomas 5-6-99

WHERE IS HE?

Where is the wonderful man I married?

Where is his gentle voice of re-assurance?

His warm tender touch that made me feel all is well,

His shoulder that comforted me when I was sad or hurt.

Where is he?

My wonderful husband I have loved for so many years.

I yearn to have him say "You are all I have ever wanted."

I yearn for the unselfish person he was.

I yearn for his discussions of dreams we shared.

And our yearly goals that made us look forward to the
    coming months.

Where is he?

I see his exterior being of slow movement and my heart
    aches.

I see Parkinson's Disease that has taken him from me and I
    anger.

My heart aches for there is nothing I can do to remove this
    terrible, cruel disease from him, for I would gladly take it
    to free him.

He does not understand the role I am forced to take.

Not by choice, but by need to protect him and do for him.

He is my every thought, my every prayer, that God will
    protect him and supply us with his needs.

But most of all, for God to cure him so I will never again
    have to ask,
      "Where is he?"
Written by Bette Thomas 1-27-01

One Magical Cane of Life

Walking was becoming a thing of the past,
When suddenly I saw hope that just might last.
It wasn't something I had ever seen before.
But worth a try if it would help him through a door.

Would it give me back my life partner?
This was my very hope, but could it be smarter?
The brain is not very easy to trick,
Could it be that this was a magical stick?

Excitement soared through me as going home I prayed,
"Please let this be not another rejection in the way!"
As my Parkinson's partner gazed at this thing,
He said, "What now did you today bring?"

With doubts he said, "I'll try it and see if it works."
Like magic he walked through doorway after doorway.

And since that day, he has not stumbled or fell to the
   floor.
Yes, this is our magical cane; the one that he will use
   forever more.

Happier than we thought we could ever be,

It gave him back once more to me you see.

My wonderful husband, cheerful and playful as a young
  boy,

For what was once despair has turned into our world of
  joy.

Written by: Bette Thomas 5-21-01

I Wonder ...?

Today, I feel so lonely. I hear no words of gratitude, no
words of thanks.

Will I ever hear them again?

I wonder ...

Am I as special as I use to be? Am I as loved as
I use to be?

Am I as comforted as I use to be?

Do I hear any kind words?

I wonder ...

The communication is so little.

The companionship of what we use to have and the despair
we now have.

PD has certainly changed our wonderful relationship
To an existence I don't like.

Will surgery give him back to me? I hope, but,
I wonder ...???

Written by: Bette Thomas 3-2-03

5

The Quality of Life Leads to Longevity

There is so much that can be done to prolong a patient's quality of life. Their Doctor can prescribe medications that help the patient maintain a normalcy of life. These medications need to be monitored every few months.

The patient needs to be encouraged to be active in activities of interest. Families can help the patient to maintain independence and freedom through encouragement.

One of the most important things you can do for the patient is to join a support group. You will meet many patients who have similar symptoms and gain a sense of togetherness in your fight to beat the illness your patient is suffering with. Support Groups will help relieve stress and help families to realize they are not alone.

The busier the patient is kept doing things he/she likes, the longer they will live a good quality of life.

6

Adult Day Care Centers

Day Care offers a wide variety of services and programs for the patient who needs care during the day. Some of the services are medication dispensing, door to door transportation, individual care plans, and blood pressure checks. Not all of the services are offered at all centers.

All medications must be in the prescription bottle with patients name, dosage, and times to be taken. Most centers keep medications in a locked cabinet. They despense the medications according to the bottle directions.

Door to door transportation is offered for a nominal fee unless the patient is a Medicaid recipient. Your Day Care Centers can supply you with correct information regarding transportation.

While the patient is at the center, they receive a hot breakfast and lunch. They also give them 2 snacks. All meals are well balanced and nutritious. They provide exercise and assistance with activities of daily living.

Some of the activities they provide are arts and crafts, bingo, other games, and puzzles. They also have daily devotions, movies, sing-a-longs, and holiday celebrations. Most centers provide a small area for those who like gardens.

Day Care gives the caregiver a respite time for personal appointments. I found Day Care to be a life saver when the patient can no longer be left alone.

Every state has different laws and facilities so it is a good idea to check with your state's recommended rules and laws. I would also like to recommend that you check with your attorney regarding Medicaid laws in your area.

If you are unable to get Day Care help, you might try your Local Home Health Service as well as Senior Centers. They can suggest other agencies to check into.

7

Nursing Home

As I am sure you all know, Nursing Homes are very expensive. They can deplete a life savings in a short time span. They are a necessity to every community. If you feel you will be needing one in the near future, by all means, get your patient's name on their waiting list. Also, check into their rules and laws for eligibility and how their payments are to be paid.

Visit as many Nursing Homes in your area and ask questions regarding their care of the patients. Check into the meals they serve the patients.

8

Hospice

I had a misconception of thoughts about what Hospice was all about until I asked a team to come and speak to my caregiver's group. The team consists of a nurse, clergy or counselor, social worker, and well trained volunteers. Their goal is to help keep the patient as pain free as possible. They will assess the patient and develop a plan that meets the needs of a pain free goal for that patient. The patient's doctor is always involved in the plans for the patient.

Hospice works closely with family and friends of the patient. The natural course of the patients disease process allows for his/her life to be enhanced with Hospice workers compassion and dignity. For the patient and loved ones, Hospice provides counseling services.

Donations to Hospice is one source of monetary funds for them to carry on their wonderful work. Many times this comes by way of the passing of a patient. The family asks for donations to be sent instead of flowers. If you want more information about Hospice, by all means, contact them. You will be pleasantly surprised at the wonderful work they do in your community.

9

Grieving Process

Grieving is a natural process in which everyone goes through differently. There are many ways to grieve. Some people cry at every mention of their loved one's name. Crying releases the stress they feel. Others may not be able to focus nor stay focused. Even though the caregiver may have the patients Advanced Directives, he/she may feel a lot of guilt when instructing a doctor of the patient's wishes. Some feel numbness as if in a cloud that keeps following them.

How long one grieves is up to the individual and is as long as it takes to adjust to the changes in your life.

Conclusion

I was the caregiver for my husband and became frustrated when he had trouble with dressing, eating, and all aspects of every day living. I knew there had to be answers for all the problems he was encountering. No one seemed to address these issues. Being just satisfied was not for me. I began to search for solutions to the problems. I was determined that others would be able to have this information that I had accumulated over the passed 31 years. This book became my dream of helping others with these daily struggles and thus, easing their pain and despair.

Resources for Further Reading

I'll Hold Your Hand So You Won't Fall. By: Rasheda Ali

The Power of Positive Thinking. By: Norman Vincint Peale

We Are Not Alone-Learning to Cope With Chronic Illness. By: Sefra Kobrin Pitzele

Peace, Love, and Healing. By: Bernie Siegel, M. D.

The Man Who Mistook His Wife for a Hat & Other Clinical Tales. By: Oliver Sacks

Mainstay. By: Maggie Strong

The 36-Hour Day. By: Nancy L. Mace & Peter V. Rabins, M. D.

Head First. By: Norman Cousins

Anatomy of an Illness. By: Norman Cousins

Parkinson's Disease Medications Book. By: Jean Hubble, M. D. and Richard Berchou, Pharm. D.

My Fading Full Moon: A Husband Journal. By: Boen Hallum

Sex, Love, and Chronic Illness. By Lucille Carlton

Parkinson's Disease: The Mystery, The Search, and The Promise. By: Sue Dauphin

More Living With Parkinson's Disease: A Patient's Perspective or I Aint Down Yet—

I'm Still Blinkin By: Jon Robert Peirce

Parkinson's: A Patient's View. By: Sidney Dorros

Living Well With Parkinson's By: Glenna Wooten Atwood

Caring for the Parkinson Patient. By: J. Thomas Hutton, M.D. & Raye L. Dipple, M. D.

Parkinson's Disease. By: Roger C. Duvoisin, M. D.

"Movement Disorders." By: Official Journal of the Movement Disorder Society.

Vol. 4/Supplement 1/1989

My Love, My Care, My Spouse. By: Eva B. Popper

From Rage to Courage. By: Michel Monnet

The Parkinson Handbook. By: Dwight C. McGoon, M. D.

When Bad Things Happen to Good People. By: Harold S. Kushner

Living With Parkinson's Disease or Don't Rush Me! I'm Coping As Fast As I Can. By: Jon Robert Pierce

Parkinson's, A Personal Story of Acceptance. By: Sandi Gordon

Courage Behind the Mask: Coping With Parkinson's Disease. By: Lucille Carlton & Dr. Robert E. Carlton

Medical Catalogs:

<u>Sammons Preston</u> (Ability One) Call 1-800-323-5547

<u>Dr. Leonards Catalog</u> (Free) Call 1-800-785-0880

<u>National Foundation of (name of Illness)</u> They will be happy to send you free booklets.

Qualifying Statement

Learn how to extend your patient's life and allow he/she to be more independent.

My caregiving experience has been taking care of my spouse for 31 years. It is through this experience that I saw a need to get information to other caregivers there-by making their job easier and less stressful. I am presently The Caregiver Leader for our Support Group in Lexington, Kentucky.

978-0-595-42617-.
0-595-42617-4

www.ingramcontent.com/pod-product-compliance
Lightning Source LLC
Chambersburg PA
CBHW050345290526
45785CB00006B/2638